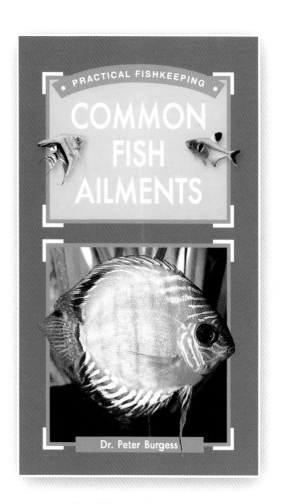

PRACTICAL FISHKEEPING

COMMON FISH AILMENTS

Dr. Peter Burgess

Dr. Peter Burgess

RINGPRESS

ABOUT THE AUTHOR

Dr. Peter Burgess is an experienced aquarium hobbyist and fish health scientist, having researched fish diseases for his MSc and PhD degrees. He is a visiting lecturer in Aquarium Sciences at the University of Plymouth, England, and edits the international science journal *Aquarium Sciences and Conservation*.

Among his other roles, Dr. Burgess is Senior Consultant to Aquarian® fishfoods and provides a fish health advisory service to ornamental fish traders and fish farms worldwide. He regularly writes for *Practical Fishkeeping* magazine.

Commercial products shown in this book are for illustrative purposes only and are not necessarily endorsed by the author.

Photography: *Dr Peter Burgess (p.11, p.14, p.24, p.25, p.27, p.29, p.37, p.39, p.40, p.45, p.46, p.47, p.48, p.52, p.54, p.55, p.56, p.57); Mary Bailey (p.26, p.38, p.41); Mike Sandford (p.44)*
Line drawings: *Viv Rainsbury*
Picture editor: *Claire Horton-Bussey*
Design: *Rob Benson*

**Published by Ringpress Books,
a division of Interpet Publishing,
Vincent Lane, Dorking, Surrey, RH4 3YX, UK
Tel: 01306 873822   Fax: 01306 876712
email: sales@interpet.co.uk**

First published 2002
© 2002 Ringpress Books. All rights reserved

ISBN 1 86054 250 6

Printed and bound in Hong Kong through Printworks International Ltd.

10 9 8 7 6 5 4 3 2 1

CONTENTS

CHAPTER
1

CREATING A HEALTHY ENVIRONMENT

Many fishkeepers only start to read up about fish health problems when actually confronted with dead or dying specimens. This is regrettable, as most common fish ailments are easily prevented by following a few simple rules.

If you familiarise yourself with the basics of fish health and aquarium management, you will avoid wasting money on medications and replacing lost stocks. But far more importantly, you will be able to offer the fish in your aquarium a long and healthy life.

THE DEMANDS WE MAKE
Compared with fish living in the wild, aquarium fish are typically kept in large numbers in confined conditions. Inevitably, this makes the aquarium a fragile environment as a lot of fish must survive

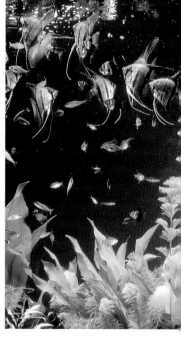

Aquarium hygiene is an essential factor in the prevention of disease.

together in a small volume of water. The fishkeeper must therefore carefully manage the aquarium or it will quickly become polluted, causing major problems to its inhabitants. There are two major areas of concern: keeping the aquarium clean and maintaining the correct water conditions.

KEEPING CLEAN

There is no escape for fish in an aquarium – they cannot swim away when conditions become unhealthy, they have to exist in the conditions you have created.

The first problem to confront is fish waste. Fish produce both solid wastes (faeces) and soluble wastes (excreted as urine and via the gills) which are passed into the water. To put it crudely, fish have to live in their own loo! To make matters worse, snails, plants and other living organisms that share the fish's aquarium will also generate wastes in the form of faeces, dead leaves and tiny decomposing bodies.

If this situation was allowed to continue unchecked, these waste substances would reach concentrations that would harm or even kill the fish. Large amounts of organic waste matter in the aquarium can also serve as a breeding ground for harmful bacteria.

It is perfectly normal for an aquarium to contain small amounts of decomposing wastes. The key to good aquarium management is to avoid excessive quantities of wastes from accumulating. This can be achieved through filtration and regular aquarium maintenance.

UNDERSTANDING FILTRATION

Fish produce ammonia as a waste product, which is excreted into the water mostly via their gills. Ammonia

CAUSES AND CONSEQUENCES OF DIRTY AQUARIUM CONDITIONS

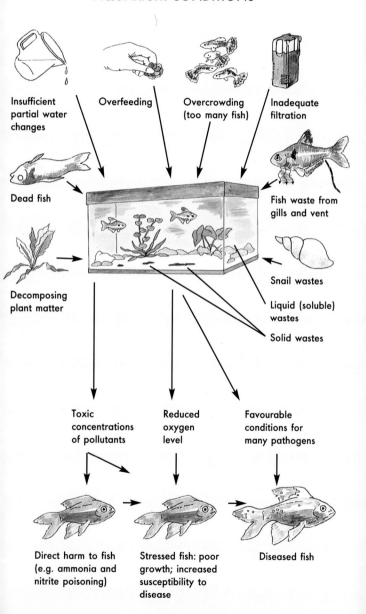

in the water is highly toxic to fish – even low levels can cause gill and skin damage. Fortunately, various types of 'friendly' bacteria naturally inhabit the aquarium and these break down ammonia into nitrite which is less toxic, and finally into relatively harmless nitrate. The role of a biological filter is to provide suitable conditions for vast numbers of these friendly 'nitrifying' bacteria.

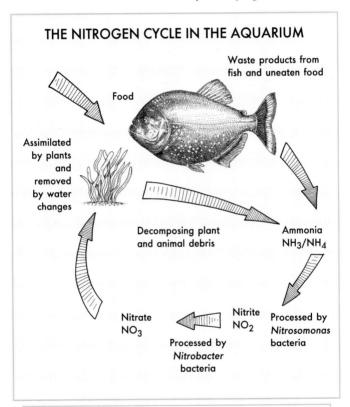

THE NITROGEN CYCLE IN THE AQUARIUM

Waste products from fish and uneaten food

Food

Assimilated by plants and removed by water changes

Decomposing plant and animal debris

Ammonia NH_3/NH_4

Nitrate NO_3

Processed by *Nitrobacter* bacteria

Nitrite NO_2

Processed by *Nitrosomonas* bacteria

DID YOU KNOW?
The ammonia wastes produced by fish are invisible and undetectable by smell, so the aquarium water can be crystal clear yet deadly to its inhabitants.

ESSENTIAL CHECKS

Ideally, the aquarium water should always have undetectable levels of ammonia and nitrite, indicating that the biological filter is functioning properly and coping with all the fish's wastes. The end product of biological filtration is nitrate which will gradually accumulate in the water. Low levels of nitrate are safe and normal, but when the level exceeds 70 mg per litre this can actually harm fish by inhibiting their growth and making them prone to diseases. The nitrate level must therefore be kept in check by performing regular, partial water changes (see page 10).

ACTION PLAN

Organic wastes	Maximum recommended level (mg/L)*	Action to take if level exceeeds recommended maximum
Ammonia	0.2**	Without delay: undertake one or more partial (25-50%) water changes until a safe level is reached.
Nitrite	0.5	Investigate the underlying cause – e.g. filter may be blocked or inadequate for the number of fish. Overfeeding and overcrowding may also be responsible.
Nitrate	70	Perform regular partial water changes.

* mg/L = milligrams per litre (= parts per million, or ppm)

** expressed as total ammonia (as measured by most aquarium test kits)

It is a good idea to routinely test for ammonia, nitrite and nitrate every week, and take the appropriate action detailed below. Ammonia and nitrite testing is particularly important when the aquarium is first set up (i.e. until the filter matures). See water test kits, page 13.

GOOD HOUSEKEEPING
Controlling waste is the key to good aquarium hygiene. This is achieved in several ways:

1. Ensure the aquarium is adequately filtered
All aquariums should be fitted with a filter. Most filters act both mechanically (removing fish faeces) and biologically (harbouring beneficial bacteria that break down poisonous wastes). In terms of fish health, the filter's biological function is more important than its mechanical role, and these filters are usually described as 'biological filters' or simply 'bio-filters'. (Your aquarium dealer can show you a range of bio-filter models to suit your size of aquarium and can explain how to service them.)

2. Do not overfeed your fish
Overfeeding is a common mistake among novice fishkeepers. As a general rule, feed little and often, perhaps two to three times each day, giving only as much food as the fish will consume within five minutes. Uneaten food will decompose and may cause a pollution problem.

3. Do not overcrowd the aquarium
Too many fish will result in large amounts of fish wastes that can overwhelm the bio-filter.

4. Perform regular partial water changes

These will remove soluble wastes. As a rule, siphon out 20-25 per cent of the aquarium water every couple of weeks, replacing it with dechlorinated tap water that has been adjusted to aquarium temperature. By fitting a gravel cleaner attachment to the siphon tube, the routine partial water change can additionally help to reduce the amounts of solid wastes within the substrate.

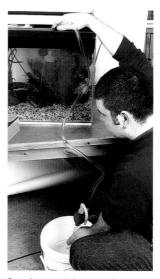

Regular, partial water changes using a siphon tube with gravel cleaner attachment remove soluble and solid wastes from the tank.

WATER CONDITIONS

The vast majority of fishkeepers use domestic tap water for filling the aquarium. Tap water must be dechlorinated (see page 12) and adjusted to aquarium temperature before adding to the tank.

The chemical composition of tap water will vary considerably between regions. It is influenced by the local geology, the lie of the land, and other factors. For example, water that has run through lime-bearing rocks will be high in certain minerals and is termed 'hard'. Fortunately, many popular aquarium fishes tolerate of a wide range of tap water conditions; however, some species have special requirements and may die if they are not provided with water of suitable chemical composition. The most important considerations are:

TEMPERATURE

Most tropical aquarium fish require a water
temperature somewhere within the range 21 to 26°C
(70 to 79°F). Aquarium heater-thermostats are factory-
set at about 24°C (75°F) and this temperature suits
most species.

pH

This is a measurement of the acidity or alkalinity of
water. The pH scale runs from 0 (extremely acid) to
14 (extremely alkaline). The mid-value, pH 7, is termed
neutral. Most tropical aquarium fish require a pH
within the region 6.6 to 7.8. (Note: pH is usually
quoted to one decimal place.)

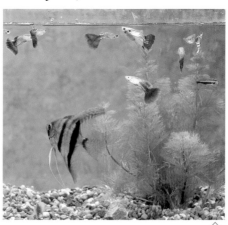

Most common
aquarium fish
are tolerant of a
wide range of
tap water
conditions but
there are many
exceptions.

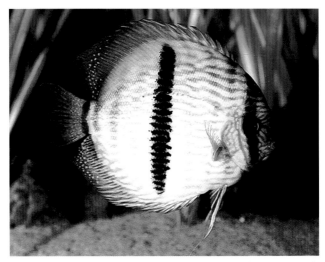

Some tropical fish, such as the South American discus (*Symphysodon*), require soft-water conditions.

HARDNESS

This is a measurement of the amount of minerals dissolved in the water, principally calcium and magnesium salts. Water is termed 'soft' or 'hard' depending on whether it is low or high in minerals, respectively. Most aquarium fish tolerate moderately hard or soft conditions, but a few require extremes of hardness or softness. As a general rule, soft waters tend to be acid, and hard waters alkaline.

Warning: do not use water that has been softened with a commercial water softener (i.e. the type installed for domestic use, which exchanges calcium for sodium ions), as it is harmful to fish.

TAP WATER AND CHLORINE

Chlorine is added to tap water to make it safe for human consumption. However, this disinfectant is potentially lethal to fish, harming their gills and skin.

Tap water must be de-chlorinated before it can be added to the aquarium. This is achieved by pre-mixing the tap water with a few drops of dechlorinator reagent (available under various brand names from the aquarium store). Alternatively, tap water can be vigorously aerated (using an airpump and an airstone) for a few hours in a clean bucket or other suitable container in order to expel the chlorine.

Note: some water supply companies use a more persistent form of chlorine, known as chloramine, to disinfect tap water – in which case you will need to use a dechlorinator reagent that removes both chloramine and chlorine. It's best to play safe and use this "dual-purpose" dechlorinator in all situations.

WATER TEST KITS

The pH, hardness, ammonia, nitrite and nitrate levels of the aquarium water can each be measured using simple test kits that can be obtained from the aquarium store. Most tests are based on a simple colour change reaction, so it is easy to read the results. As an alternative to buying your own test kits, some aquarium stores offer a water-testing service for a small fee.

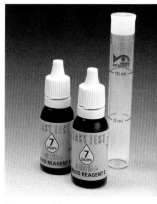

Water test kits can measure a host of different chemical levels in the aquarium water.

OTHER CONSIDERATIONS

A well-managed aquarium with the correct water conditions will give your fish every chance of living a healthy life. However, there are other points to consider:

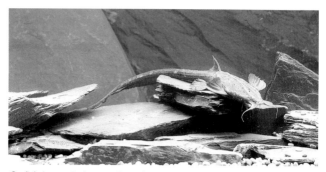
Catfish in particular require substrate and decor at the bottom of the tank in order to feel secure.

STOCKING DENSITY
This is the quantity of fish that an aquarium can safely accommodate. The fish-carrying capacity of an aquarium is mostly dictated by its surface area (see page 60 for calculations). Overcrowding can lead to pollution, stress and disease outbreaks. Before choosing fish, find out how large they will grow.

COMPATIBILITY
Choose species that will live in relative harmony.

TYPE AND QUANTITY OF DECOR
Bare tanks will cause stress to most fish, and they cannot thrive if the habitat provided is unsuitable. Some species require rock caves to hide in, others may prefer densely planted aquariums in order to feel secure. Find out what suits the fish you are planning to keep before designing your aquarium.

CHAPTER 2

UNDERSTANDING DISEASE

Diseases can be classified as 'non-infectious' or 'infectious', and it is obviously important to recognise which category a disease falls into in order to take the appropriate measures.

NON-INFECTIOUS DISEASES

These include conditions such as chemical poisoning (e.g. due to water pollution or incorrect water conditions); injuries; body abnormalities (e.g. organ failure, perhaps due to old age), and nutritional deficiencies (e.g. resulting from an inadequate or incorrect diet).

Although these conditions cannot spread from fish to fish, some of these diseases (notably those caused by adverse water conditions) can harm most, or all, the fish within an aquarium.

INFECTIOUS DISEASES

These are caused by various types of organisms: viruses, bacteria, fungi and parasites (page 16). Infectious diseases can spread from fish to fish, sometimes quite rapidly, and some affect a wide range of fish species.

FISHKEEPING TIP
Buy a quality hand lens (magnifying glass) for close inspection of your fish for signs of disease.

Group	Size	Occurrence of the fish	Disease example
MAJOR GROUPS OF INFECTIOUS DISEASE ORGANISMS			
Pathogens			
Viruses	Sub-microscopic. Visible only with a special 'electron microscope'	Varies according to the type of virus. As a group, viruses can affect most organs, internal or external	Lympho-cystis
Bacteria	Microscopic	Varies according to the bacteria species. As a group, they can affect most organs, internal or external	Ulcers Fin-rot Dropsy
Fungi	Colonies of fungi are generally visible to the naked eye	Almost always on the body surface	Fungus disease
Parasites			
Protozoa	Vast majority are micro-scopic. A few are just visible to the naked eye or with a hand lens	Varies according to protozoan species. As a group they can affect most organs, internal or external. Several commonly encountered species live on or just under the skin	White-spot
Leeches	Large parasites, visible to the naked eye	Attach to the skin or gills	Not common in tropical aquarium
Crusta-ceans	Many are visible to the naked eye	Most attach to the skin or gills.	Not common in tropical aquarium

Nema-tode worms (round-worms)	Many are large but remain out-of-sight within the fish's body	Internal. Most live within the fish's gut	Not commonly detected in tropical aquarium fish
Flukes	Some are just visible with a hand lens	Commonly encountered species live on the skin and/or gills. Others live as relatively harmless larval stages beneath the skin or in the muscles and organs	Certain forms of skin irritation (caused by skin flukes). Certain respiratory problems (caused by gill flukes)
Tape-worms	Many are large but remain out-of-sight within the fish's body	Internal. Adult tapeworms live within the fish's gut. Larval stages occur in the body cavity	Not commonly detected in tropical aquarium fish

Note: although most disease organisms cannot be seen by the naked eye, the diseases they cause often show as visible outward signs on the fish, such as spots, lumps, ulcers, haemorrhages and so on.

PREVENTING INFECTIOUS DISEASES

The first consideration is to minimise the likelihood of introducing disease-causing organisms (pathogens and parasites) into the aquarium. Various routes by which these undesirable organisms may enter an aquarium are shown in the illustration on page 18.

Fish and their transport water (i.e. the water in which they are bagged) are the most likely source of pathogens and parasites.

HOW PATHOGENS AND PARASITES CAN ENTER AN AQUARIUM

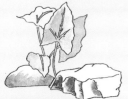

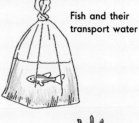

Fish and their transport water

Live plants and unwashed rocks collected from natural waters or ornamental ponds, or from another (diseased) aquarium or pond

Certain wild-collected live foods, e.g. *Tubifex* worms

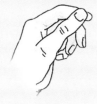

Unwashed hands that have recently been immersed in another (diseased) aquarium or pond

Nets and other equipment (heaters, filters, etc.) recently used in another (diseased) aquarium

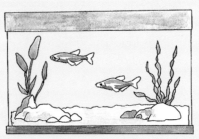

All the above are common routes of entry.

It is extremely unlikely that pathogens or parasites could enter the aquarium via tapwater, the air or dry formulation fish foods (e.g. flakes, pellets).

The risk of bringing in infectious diseases via new fish can be greatly reduced by taking a few precautions:

- Purchase fish from a reputable supplier, ideally a specialist aquarium store.
- When selecting fish for purchase, inspect *all* the fish within the aquarium (see page 21 for signs of a healthy fish). If the aquarium houses dead, dying, or diseased fish, then do not make a purchase, even if the particular specimen(s) that you have selected appear healthy – they could be incubating a disease, or there could be pathogens in the water (most pathogens are microscopic so you will not see them).
- If possible, quarantine newly-purchased fish before introducing them to your main aquarium. A quarantine period of two weeks is recommended. During this time, closely monitor the fish for any signs of disease, and treat where necessary.

LIVE FOODS AND DISEASE

Certain live fish foods, notably *Tubifex* worms, may harbour fish pathogens, so feeding them to fish carries a significant degree of risk. Other popular live foods, such as *Daphnia* ('water fleas'), mosquito larvae, and bloodworms (fly larvae) are far less risky. Safer still are the frozen, gamma-irradiated forms of these live foods which are sold in foil or blister packs (these foods must be stored in a freezer until ready to feed).

THE QUARANTINE AQUARIUM

Where possible, all newly-purchased fish should be quarantined for 10-14 days. A five-gallon aquarium (20-25 litres) is usually adequate for all but the largest fish. Several fish can be quarantined together, provided they are compatible with each other and the tank is large enough to accommodate them all.

Rocks and other decor should be kept to a minimum – just enough to make the fish feel at ease. Use plastic plants instead of live ones, as they can be washed afterwards.

There is no need for an aquarium light, but do provide heat (a 50-watt heater-thermostat is adequate for a five-gallon tank) and filtration. An electrically operated canister filter (with sponge cartridge) or air-driven box filter (containing synthetic filter medium) is generally suitable.

TIPS FOR QUARANTINING FISH

- **Feed sparingly during quarantine, to minimise pollution.**
- **Maintain optimal water conditions. Perform a 20 per cent water change once or twice a week. Check ammonia and nitrite levels every few days.**
- **Monitor the fish during quarantine. Do not add medications unnecessarily – only if a disease occurs (in which case remove any activated carbon from the filter, otherwise it will absorb the medication).**
- **You can dismantle the aquarium after use. Rinse and dry the decor and equipment, and store it until needed again.**
- **Use the quarantine tank and equipment solely for quarantine purposes.**
- **The quarantine aquarium can also be used to isolate and medicate fish that have fallen ill in the main aquarium.**

The filter is unlikely to be biologically mature, so add some zeolite (from the aquarium store) to the filter chamber to absorb ammonia wastes. Replenish the zeolite periodically (see the manufacturer's instructions). Never use zeolite in conjunction with a salt treatment.

SIGNS OF GOOD HEALTH

Get into the habit of routinely checking the health of your fish. A healthy fish:

- Does not repeatedly scratch its body on objects.
- Does not gasp at the surface.
- In the case of shoaling species: a healthy fish will swim with the main group.
- Exhibits a normal respiratory rate (see page 49, Respiration in fish).
- Readily takes food.

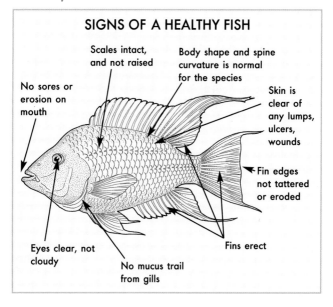

SIGNS OF A HEALTHY FISH

Scales intact, and not raised

Body shape and spine curvature is normal for the species

No sores or erosion on mouth

Skin is clear of any lumps, ulcers, wounds

Fin edges not tattered or eroded

Eyes clear, not cloudy

No mucus trail from gills

Fins erect

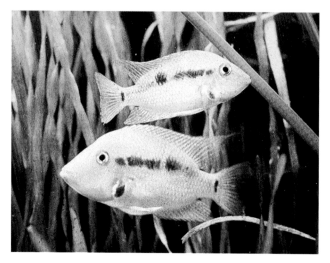

Stressed fish lose coloration. Pictured: *Thorichthys meeki* (Firemouth Cichlid) kept under unsuitable conditions and showing none of their characteristic orange–red coloration.

Some species of fish deviate from the 'norm' and look or behave in ways that could be misinterpreted as unhealthy. For example, botias (a type of loach) may lie on their sides when resting, and certain African *Synodontis* catfish naturally swim upside-down! At spawning time, some types of fish (e.g. cichlids) exhibit changes in their behaviour, coloration and body markings, and some hide away to guard eggs or fry.

As you gain familiarity with individual fish species, you will be able to distinguish between normal and abnormal (unhealthy) behaviour.

STRESS-RELATED PROBLEMS

In the wild, stress has a natural and sometimes beneficial role to play in the life of fish (indeed for any animal). In captivity, however, where fish are relatively crowded and confined within a small space, extremely stressful situations may arise that can adversely affect

CAUSES OF STRESS IN AQUARIUM FISH

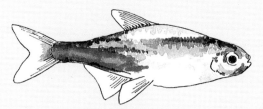

UNSTRESSED FISH

Water pollution →   ← Overcrowding

Incorrect water conditions →

     ← Bullying or fighting

Transportation (recently →
introduced fish)

     ← Inadequate décor
     (e.g. bare tank)

Incorrect water →
temperature (too low;
too high)

     ← Repeated disturbance
     from outside (e.g.
     children banging on
     glass)

Frequent re-arrangement →
of décor (fish prefer to
have stable and familiar
surroundings)

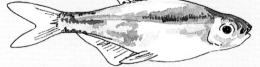

STRESSED FISH

Prolonged stress makes the fish prone to disease

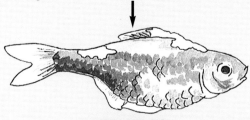

DISEASED FISH

the fish's health. Highly stressed fish are prone to infectious diseases and other health problems.

Unfortunately, no aquarium can ever be totally stress-free. However, the aquarist should try to prevent highly stressful conditions from occurring. Common stressors (i.e. things that cause stress) affecting aquarium fish are shown in the panel on page 23.

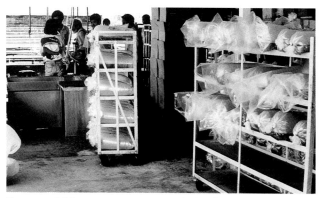

Transported fish are prone to stress, and, therefore, to disease. Pictured: fish bagged up for export.

TRANSPORTATION STRESS

Recently-imported fish are very likely to be stressed as a result of having been transported (often for thousands of miles) under crowded and confined conditions. Not surprisingly, such fish are prone to disease outbreaks, which is why aquarium stores should quarantine new stock before offering them for sale.

CHAPTER
3

THE FISH HEALTH DETECTIVE

Investigating the cause of an illness or death usually requires an element of detective work. In some cases, the problem will always remain a mystery, despite all efforts to locate the cause. The golden rule is to act as soon as a problem arises – never wait for the fish to get worse or for more fish to die.

READING THE CLUES
The following three scenarios are intended to help you track down the cause of a fish health problem.

> **1. A newly purchased fish becomes ill or dies within a few days after being introduced to the aquarium**

This scenario assumes that the established fish (i.e. those that have been resident in the aquarium for several weeks or more) appeared healthy at the time the new fish was introduced.

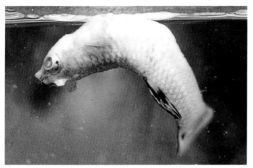

A number of factors could be responsible for the death of a new fish.

- Is the fish suited to your aquarium's water conditions (notably temperature and pH)? Test the water conditions to ensure they are within acceptable limits.
- Could the fish have died from nitrate shock (check the nitrate level of your water – it should be less than 70 mg/L)? Deaths due to nitrate shock often occur between 24 and 72 hours after introduction.
- The fish may have died from poisoning (see page 29)
- The fish may have been ill or incubating a disease prior to purchase. Did it appear healthy when you acquired it? Does the fish display any visible disease signs? Keep a close check on your other fish in case the disease is infectious.
- The fish may have been attacked by its new tankmates. This is not uncommon with certain types of fish, such as cichlids. Consider whether the new fish is socially compatible with your existing stock.
- Could the fish have been traumatised during the journey home? Perhaps the transport container became too hot or too cold? Never delay in getting the fish home once purchased.

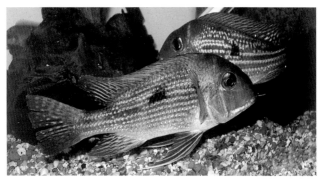

A *Geophagus* cichlid with a split and frayed tail, probably caused by aggression.

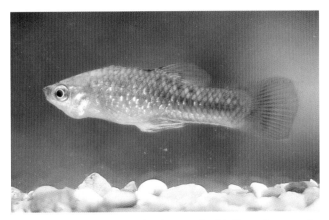
Sometimes old age is responsible for poor health. Pictured: an aged livebearer, with a sunken belly and clamped fins.

2. A single established fish becomes ill or dies

This scenario relates to a fish that has been resident in the aquarium for several weeks or more. The other fish in the aquarium appear healthy.

- The fish may have been attacked or killed by another fish. Certain types of fish (e.g. cichlids and some gouramis) may become particularly aggressive at spawning time, attacking their spawning partner or other fish entering their breeding territory.
- Old age. Some fish live for only a year or two.
- Adverse water conditions. The aquarium water conditions may have changed or deteriorated such that they are no longer tolerated by the affected fish, but may still be within the tolerance limits of its tankmates. Check the water conditions in the aquarium.

FISHKEEPING TIP
Isolate a sick fish wherever possible (page 19) – just in case it is suffering from an infectious disease.

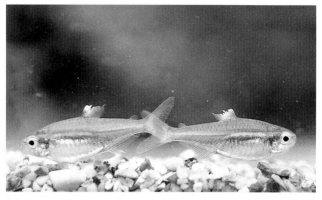

Injuries can be sustained from décor, handling or fighting. Pictured: Glowlight Tetras with cropped dorsal fins caused by fin-nipping.

- Injury from recent clumsy handling (e.g. the fish jumped out of a net and on to the floor).
- Injury from fighting, or damage from décor (e.g. sharp rocks).
- The fish may be suffering from a pathogen or parasite problem. Are there any obvious disease symptoms? If you suspect a disease, then closely monitor your other fish over the next few weeks in case it is infectious.

3. Multiple sudden deaths of established stock

If several previously healthy fish die within a brief time span (i.e within a 48-hour period), this is most likely to be a water problem. Very few infectious diseases will kill previously healthy fish so quickly. Check the water conditions, especially ammonia, nitrite, pH and temperature.

Note: a very dirty or overcrowded aquarium can cause sudden multiple deaths due to a rapid fall in the dissolved oxygen level. Fish that have died of oxygen starvation often have their mouths wide open and gill covers flared.

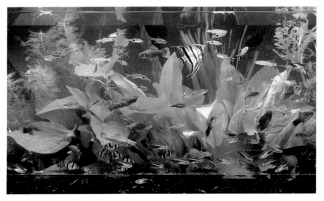

An overcrowded aquarium can be a killer, so ensure the tank is large enough to house the size and number of fish you wish to keep.

POISONS AND POLLUTANTS

The aquarist may discover that some or all of his fish are dying for no apparent reason. When there are no visible signs of infection or injuries and no obvious water-quality problems, occasionally these 'mystery' fish deaths are due to poisoning.

'Natural' poisons, such as ammonia and nitrite, have already been discussed (pages 7-9). Other poisons can enter the aquarium via the air or by leaching from aquarium rocks or other contaminated décor (see table, page 18).

Depending on the nature and concentration of the poison, the effects on fish may be acute or chronic:

FISHKEEPING TIP

If a fish dies (for whatever reason), remove the corpse without delay, as corpses can pollute the water and may harbour pathogens. If you plan to submit the corpse to a vet for a postmortem, store it in a plastic bag and put it in the fridge, but never the freezer, as freeze-thawing will render it useless for postmortem.

- **Acute poisoning:** Sickness or deaths occur over a few hours, or even minutes, often involving a complete wipe-out of all fish. This can happen, for example, if the fish are accidentally exposed to heavily chlorinated tap water or bleach (both rapidly harm their gills).

- **Chronic poisoning:** Sickness or deaths may occur over a prolonged period of time, with perhaps just one or two fish dying every few days. This can arise from a gradual accumulation of the poison within the aquarium water (e.g. the slow leaching of poisonous metal salts from a rock). Fish vary in their sensitivity to poisons, hence some will be affected sooner than others.

Many common poisons affect the fish's gills or nervous system, causing respiratory problems or skittish and uncoordinated swimming behaviour, respectively.

Note: many chemicals that poison fish are both colourless and odourless, so their presence in the aquarium may not be obvious.

DOMESTIC CLEANING AGENTS
Soaps, detergents and bleaches are all potentially toxic to fish, even in trace amounts, causing gill damage and other problems, sometimes death.

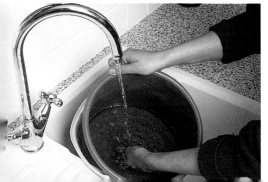

A bucket assigned only for aquarium use will prevent potentially toxic cleaning agents from being introduced to the fish unwittingly when cleaning gravel or adding water to the tank.

- When filling/emptying aquariums, avoid using 'household' buckets that may have held cleaning agents. Play safe and purchase a new plastic bucket and label it 'for aquarium use only'.
- Rinse hands free of soap before immersing them into an aquarium.
- Never use these cleaning agents to wash gravel, decor, filter medium, or other materials used in the aquarium. Most aquarium equipment can be satisfactorily cleaned using tap water only.

HARMFUL FUMES AND AEROSOLS

These air-borne poisons can enter the aquarium water via the surface (paint and varnish fumes may form a cloudy surface film or scum), or be drawn into the aquarium via the air-pump.

Gloss paint and varnish fumes are potentially harmful to fish, and, for this reason, the aquarium should be temporarily relocated before undertaking major decorating work using these materials.

Avoid using aerosol fly-killers and other insecticide sprays near the aquarium, as these contain pyrethroids and other substances harmful to fish. Air-fresheners may also be harmful.

FISHKEEPING TIP
If poisoning is suspected, perform a large (e.g. 75 per cent) water change without delay, ensuring that the replacement water is dechlorinated and matched for temperature and pH. Repeat 24 to 48 hours later. Track down and eliminate the cause of poisoning.

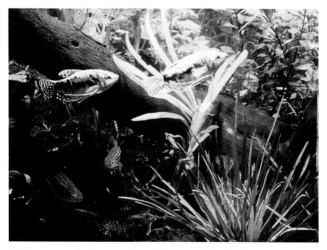

Unlike many other types of wood, bogwood bought from an aquarium store will not introduce harmful pollutants to your tank.

AQUARIUM DECOR

Aquarium décor includes gravel, rocks, wood, ornaments, aquatic plants (live or artificial) and other under-water furnishings. It is wise to purchase such items from the aquarium store as those sold for garden use or other purposes may be harmful to fish.

Do not collect your own rocks for aquarium use unless you are knowledgeable in geology and can identify those which are safe (inert). Never use builder's gravel or sand as they may contain harmful contaminants.

Unsupervised children have been known to drop toys or sweets into an aquarium. If necessary, fit a lock to the aquarium cover to prevent such accidents.

CHAPTER
4

COMMON FISH DISEASES

There are a number of diseases that most commonly affect tropical freshwater fish. Fortunately, several of these diseases can be successfully treated using proprietary medications (also known as disease treatments, remedies or cures) that can be purchased from most aquarium stores.

WHITESPOT DISEASE
Other common name: Ich.
Pathogen involved: *Ichthyophthirius multifiliis* (protozoan).
Typical signs: There may be few to numerous white spots on the body and/or fins, and gills. Each spot is slightly raised and up to 1 mm diameter. The number of spots on the fish may increase rapidly within a few days. It usually rapidly spreads to most or all fish.

Whitespot is a common parasitic disease of tropical freshwater fish. Numerous white spots can be seen here on the fish's fin.

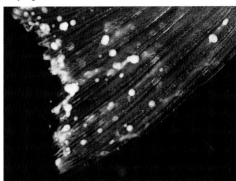

WHITESPOT LIFE CYCLE

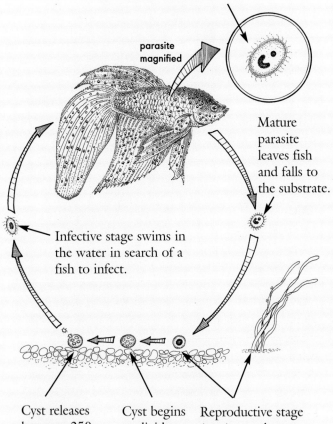

Parasitic feeding-growing stage beneath skin of fish.

parasite magnified

Mature parasite leaves fish and falls to the substrate.

Infective stage swims in the water in search of a fish to infect.

Cyst releases between 250 and 2000 infective stages.

Cyst begins to divide.

Reproductive stage (cyst) on substrate. This stage may also be found attached to plants.

Affected fish repeatedly twitch their fins and rub their flanks against rocks and other surfaces. In heavy infections, parasites on the gills may cause the fish breathing difficulties, manifesting as abnormally fast gill beats, and the fish may hang near the water surface.

In severe cases, the fish's skin may slough away in patches. Parasite damage to the skin renders the fish susceptible to fungal and bacterial infections.

Causes: The most likely source of whitespot is via recently-introduced fish. Small numbers of parasites on newly-purchased fish are not easily detected (especially on pale-skinned specimens), and microscopic free-living stages may be present in the fish's transport water.

Treatment: Proprietary whitespot remedies are generally very effective. One or two repeat treatments are usually necessary in order to completely eradicate whitespot from the aquarium – see manufacturer's instructions regarding re-dosing. It is important to treat the whole aquarium to eradicate free-living stages within the gravel and water.

Salt can be used to kill whitespot, provided *all* the fish are salt-tolerant species (seek expert advice if in doubt). Use only pure sodium chloride, never kitchen salt containing additives. Dose the aquarium with 2 grams of salt per litre, for 10 days. After this period, dilute out the salt by several partial water changes (e.g. 25 per cent every few days).

Note: treat any secondary fungal or bacterial infections, as appropriate (proprietary anti-fungus and anti-bacterial medications are widely available).

General comments: Whitespot is a common parasitic disease of freshwater fish. It is highly infectious and potentially fatal unless treated quickly.

Those fish that survive a whitespot infection may develop partial immunity to this parasite. This acquired immunity may explain why some fish that are exposed to a subsequent whitespot outbreak may harbour no or few parasites (i.e. immune fish) while others sharing the aquarium may become heavily infected and die (i.e. non-immune fish).

LYMPHOCYSTIS DISEASE
Other common name: Cauliflower disease.
Pathogen involved: *Lymphocystis* (virus).
Typical signs: One or several white, grey, or pale pink lumps on the body or fins. The lumps typically form clusters (hence 'cauliflower' disease), and vary in size from being just visible to the naked eye up to several millimetres across. The disease is chronic and the number of lumps do not increase rapidly over time. Often, only a single fish is affected (and may appear otherwise normal) and the disease is not highly contagious.

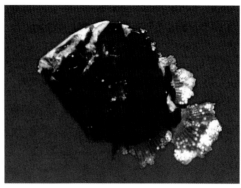

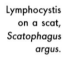
Lymphocystis on a scat, *Scatophagus argus*.

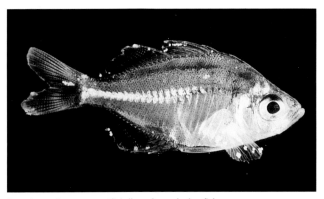
Lymphocystis on an artificially-coloured glassfish.

Causes: Many aquarium fish may harbour the virus without showing external signs of disease (i.e. no lumps). However, if these fish are stressed for any reason then the virus can become 'activated', resulting in the formation of lumps. Recently-imported fish may break out with lymphocystis due to transportation stress.

Treatment: No medications are available to combat lymphocystis or indeed any viral disease of fish. Fortunately, lymphocystis is rarely life-threatening and affected fish generally recover, if provided with optimum aquarium conditions.

Any cause of stress that may have triggered a lymphocystis outbreak in the first place must be identified and eliminated, otherwise the fish may not improve or may relapse.

General comments: Lymphocystis affects only certain types of fish – notably cichlids, gouramis (anabantids) and other evolutionary advanced groups. Conversely, it does not affect cyprinids (e.g. barbs, rasboras), tetras, or catfishes.

FUNGUS DISEASE

Other common names: Fish fungus, cotton-wool disease, saprolegnia disease.

Pathogens involved: Various aquatic fungi (=water moulds), notably *Saprolegnia* and *Achyla*.

Typical signs: Tufts of growths on the skin that resemble cotton-wool (cotton) on the fins, eyes or gills. Sometimes only a single tuft may be present, or there may be several. Each tuft is typically whitish, yellowish or pale grey, but, in time, can become dark-grey, green or red-brown (due to entrapped algae or dirt). Affected fish may appear otherwise normal. Often limited to just one fish.

Causes: Fungal spores are present in most bodies of freshwater. In most situations, fungus attacks only those tissues that have already been damaged as a result of an infection (e.g. by bacteria or skin parasites) or injury. Skin injuries caused by fighting or from rough handling are also susceptible to fungus. Fish that have a lowered immunity, perhaps due to extreme stress or from being chilled, are also at risk of fungus infections.

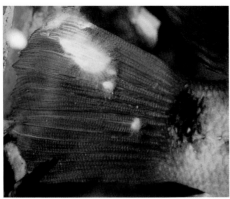

Saprolegnia on the tail.

Treatment: Proprietary anti-fungus medications are available. Because fungus is unlikely to attack healthy, undamaged fish, the affected individuals can be treated in isolation rather than medicating the whole of the aquarium.

Salt (sodium chloride), dosed at 2 grams per litre, 10 days, is also effective. See whitespot entry for further advice about salt treatments.

General comments: Try to resolve the underlying cause of the tissue damage. Failure to do so could result in renewed fungus outbreaks.

ULCER DISEASE
Other common name: Skin ulcers; sores.
Pathogens involved: Various bacteria, including *Aeromonas* spp. and *Pseudomonas* spp.
Typical signs: One or more open sores on the body. Ulcers are typically roughly circular in shape and concave (cratered). They generally have a whitish, pale pink or reddish centre, sometimes with a white or red perimeter.

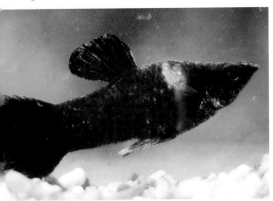

Ulcers generally have a white or pale pink centre. Pictured: ulcer on a molly.

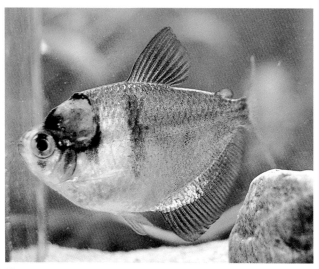

Ulcer on a black-widow tetra. Note the melanisation (blackening) around the edges.

Some skin ulcers are very deep and extend down to the underlying muscles. In some cases, just one or a few fish may develop ulcers, or several may be affected, depending on the underlying cause.

Causes: Poor aquarium hygiene, overcrowding, transportation stress, skin parasites.

Treatment: Proprietary anti-ulcer or anti-bacterial medications are sometimes effective, especially if the disease is caught at an early stage. Failing this, treatment with antibiotics will be necessary. Seek veterinary assistance regarding the selection and application of antibiotics.

General comments: Investigate any underlying cause of an ulcer outbreak, particularly unhygienic aquarium conditions.

Ulcers breach the protective skin layers, rendering the fish susceptible to other infections. Ulcerated fish should therefore be kept under hygienic conditions to improve the chances of a cure and to reduce the likelihood of secondary infections. Ulcerated fish should be moved to a clean quarantine aquarium for the duration of treatment and until the ulcers fully heal.

Extensive ulceration can upset the fish's salt balance (osmoregulation), and this, in turn, can be lethal.

FIN ROT

Other common name: Tail rot (where the tail fin is affected).

Pathogens involved: Various bacteria, notably *Flavobacterium* (formerly *Flexibacter*), *Aeromonas*, and *Pseudomonas* species.

Typical signs: Gradual disintegration of the fin, beginning with the fin becoming frayed or ragged at the outermost edge. Fin rot can affect any of the fish's fins, particularly the tail fin (caudal fin). Initially, there is a whitish (or reddish) edge to the affected fin.

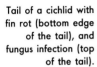

Tail of a cichlid with fin rot (bottom edge of the tail), and fungus infection (top of the tail).

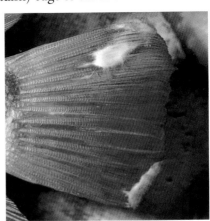

With tail rot, the infection may progress to the base of the tail and sometimes into the body tissues, resulting in a stump (at this stage the disease is often fatal). Fish suffering from severe tail rot experience difficulties in swimming, may become sluggish, and go off their food. Secondary infection with fungus can occur.

Fin rot may be limited to just one fish, in other cases many or all the fish may be involved, especially when the underlying cause is poor aquarium hygiene.

PLEASE NOTE
- If fin rot is accompanied by a swelling of the fish's body and/or bulging of its eyes, then refer to the section on Dropsy (below).
- If accompanied by ulcers on the body, then this is possibly a *Flavobacterium (Flexibacter)* infection which may respond to an anti-bacterial medication, but antibiotics are likely to be more effective.

Causes: Poor aquarium hygiene, or stress. An injury to the fin, caused by skin parasites or fin-nipping, can result in bacterial infection leading to fin rot.

Treatment: Proprietary medications are usually effective provided the infection is treated at an early stage (before progressing on to the body). Affected fish should be maintained under hygienic conditions to improve the likelihood of a cure. Any underlying cause (such as poor aquarium hygiene or fin-nipping) must be addressed in order to prevent a recurrence.

General comments: Fin rot can also occur in severe cases of whitespot disease (see page 33).

ANTIBIOTICS

These anti-bacterial substances were originally extracted from moulds and bacteria. The most famous antibiotic is Penicillin.

Antibiotics are especially useful for treating internal or stubborn bacterial infections that often do not respond to proprietary anti-bacterial medications sold in aquarium stores. Antibiotics will not cure viral diseases of fish.

Nowadays, several synthetic antibiotics are available for treating bacterial diseases of fish and each differs in terms of dosage, route of application and effectiveness. Some are effective when added to the aquarium water, but others have to be mixed with the fish's food, or given by injection (assuming the fish is large enough to be injected).

In some countries, including the UK, antibiotics can only legally be obtained by veterinary prescription. The involvement of a vet or professional fish heath scientist is, in any case, advisable so as to ensure that the most suitable antibiotic is selected and is administered in the most effective way.

Caution: some antibiotics will destroy the beneficial filter bacteria (check with your vet or fish health professional).

DROPSY (BODY SWELLING)

Other common name: Abdominal dropsy; pine cone disease.

Causes: Bacterial or viral infection, or organ failure.

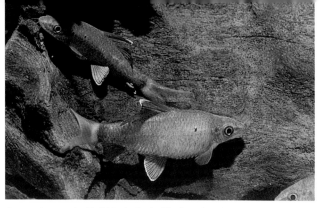

Dropsy in a red-tailed black shark (*Epalzeorhynchos bicolor*). The abdomen is swollen and the abdominal scales are projecting outwards.

Typical signs: The belly region of the fish becomes very swollen, almost spherical in some cases, due to an accumulation of fluid in the body. The scales protrude outwards to give a serrated effect to the fish's body contour – known as the 'pine cone effect' (this is more obvious when the fish is viewed from above). Often, the fish's eyes bulge ('pop-eye'). Affected fish appear very unwell, often sluggish, and off their food. It is usually fatal.

Causes: The disease is generally the result of damage to one or more internal organs that are involved in the water balance (osmoregulation) of the fish. Organ damage can itself be the result of a viral or bacterial infection or simply old age (organ failure). Poor aquarium hygiene has been implicated in some cases of dropsy.

Treatment: It is not possible to tell the cause of dropsy based on external signs alone. The best policy is to assume it is a bacterial infection and treat accordingly in the hope of effecting a cure. Unfortunately, by the time the outward symptoms have appeared the fish will already be very ill and treatment is often unsuccessful. The best hope for a cure is to treat with antibiotics.

General comments: Do not confuse dropsy with other causes of abdominal swelling. For example, female egg-laying and live-bearing fish may become swollen with eggs or fry, but, in such cases, the scales do not stick out and the fish will appear otherwise healthy.

EYE PROBLEMS

Various eye problems can occur, and each has one or more causes. Most eye problems are not highly infectious.

EYE PROTRUSION OR PROTRUDING EYE(S) (POP-EYE/EXOPHTHALMIA)

The eye(s) stick out noticeably, particularly when the fish is viewed head on, or from above. This is quite likely to be the result of an internal infection, often caused by bacteria. Eye protrusion often accompanies dropsy (see page 43), and poor aquarium hygiene is a predisposing factor.

An anti-internal bacteria medication may be effective. Alternatively, treatment with antibiotics may offer a better chance of cure, particularly if the fish also has dropsy.

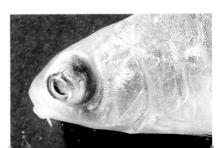

Exophthalmia (Pop-eye) is an easily-recognised condition.

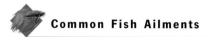

GROWTHS ON THE EYE(S)

White to grey fluffy tufts or growths may appear on one or both eyes. The eye(s) may be partly or completely covered with fungus (best seen with the aid of a magnifying lens). See Fungus diseases (page 38) for symptoms, causes and treatments.

CLOUDY EYE(S)

One or both eyes look as if they are covered by a white or semi-translucent film (which is *not* fluffy or tufted). This is likely due to a bacterial infection. It can be triggered by poor hygiene conditions or an eye injury. Treat with an anti-bacterial medication.

A less common cause of eye cloudiness is poor diet, especially if the fish has been fed on dried foods that are of poor quality or that have been improperly stored (i.e. under very warm or humid conditions) after opening. In such cases, inadequate amounts of certain vitamins in the food (notably vitamin C) can cause eye cloudiness. Always feed a high-quality dry food from a reputable manufacturer and store opened pots of food under dry, cool conditions to minimise vitamin degradation.

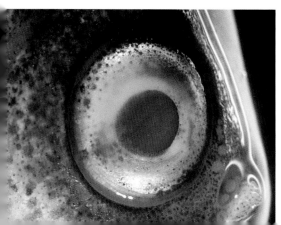

A close-up of a cloudy eye.

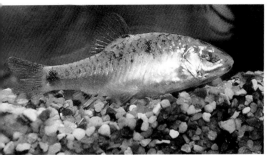

A barb with a missing eye. The socket has healed over, and the fish is otherwise healthy.

MISSING EYE(S)

Loss of one or both eyes can be due to injury, but is often the result of attack by other fish (the fins and eyes are often targeted by aggressive tankmates). If the eye socket appears infected (bloody, or exuding white matter), then treat with an anti-bacteria medication.

Most aquarium fish are not overly incapacitated by the loss of one or even both eyes, as they can often rely on other sensory systems to navigate and locate food.

RESPIRATORY PROBLEMS

Respiratory problems (fast gill beats: see box page 49) occur when the fish has difficulty in obtaining sufficient amounts of oxygen from the water. The underlying cause may be a water quality problem or gill damage.

Typical signs: Opercular (gill) beats are abnormally fast and pronounced. Affected fish may gulp at the water surface (don't confuse with surface feeding at meal-times, or normal air-gulping behaviour by fish that are able to breathe atmospheric oxygen – e.g. gouramis, fighting fish and other anabantids).

Depending on the cause, the fish may also exhibit one or more other signs of ill health: periodic coughing, unusual swimming, highly erratic or very sluggish activity, and, in some cases, flashing (page 62).

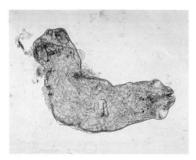

Parasites, such as the gill fluke (pictured), may be responsible for respiratory difficulties.

Causes: Respiratory distress may be due to low oxygen levels in the water or something affecting the fish's ability to take up oxygen into its tissues.

Possible causes of low oxygen levels in the water are: pollution; overcrowding; failure of the filter (perhaps blocked) or aerator. Very high water temperature, perhaps due to a faulty heater-thermostat, will reduce the oxygen level. First exclude these possibilities before considering a gill disease problem.

Damage to the fish's gills will reduce these organs' ability to take up oxygen from the water. Gill damage can be caused by chlorine (e.g. from untreated tap water) or by high levels of ammonia (e.g. resulting from inadequate biological filtration).

A high nitrite level can also cause respiratory

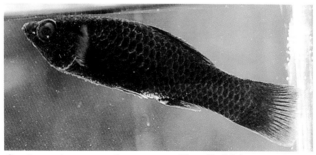

Gasping at the water surface suggests this molly fish is not receiving enough oxygen, either through poor water quality, or gill damage. Note the clamped fins — a sign of stress.

RESPIRATION IN FISH

Fish obtain oxygen from the water via their gills, these organs being analogous to the lungs of land animals. Mechanically, fish breathe by taking in water via the mouth and pumping it across the gill filaments. The dissolved oxygen is taken up across the thin gill membranes and passes into the bloodstream. The water is expelled under the gill flaps (opercula). Each 'breath' manifests as the opening and closing of the opercula, each open and close cycle being termed an 'opercular beat'. The faster the fish breathes, the higher the rate of opercular (gill) beats.

The opercular beat rate varies according to the fish species and also with water temperature (the warmer the water, the higher the rate). It will also increase during heightened activity or when the fish is frightened.

If you carefully observe a fish you can measure its opercular rate (count the number of opercular beats over a one-minute period).

Fish that are suffering from respiratory stress tend to have very fast and often pronounced opercular beats (compare with others of the same species sharing the aquarium).

problems by reducing the blood's ability to transport oxygen to the tissues. Test the water for levels of ammonia and nitrite. If the nitrite level is high, add sodium chloride (0.1 g per litre) to the aquarium water. The chloride will reduce nitrite toxicity (most fish species will tolerate this low level of salt).

If a water problem is ruled out then the fish may be suffering from gill parasites such as flukes or

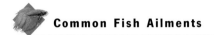

protozoans. An anti-parasite cure is worth trying in such cases. The gills can also be infected with fungus or bacteria, and should be treated accordingly using proprietary medications.

SKIN IRRITATIONS
There are many causes of skin irritation in fish, including water quality problems and skin parasites.

Typical signs: These vary according to the underlying cause, and include: fin twitching, flashing, and excess mucus production (the skin takes on a faint greyish or whitish appearance). Depending on the cause, the gills may also be affected, causing respiratory problems.

Causes: Water problems: high levels of ammonia, nitrite, or nitrate; excessively high or low pH; chlorine and chloramine; and other poisons can all cause skin irritations in fish. Hence, test the water parameters before considering the possibility of skin parasites.

Parasites: Whitespot (page 33), and various other skin-dwelling parasites may be the cause. Most skin parasites are very small and can only be properly identified with the aid of a microscope, and with a good knowledge of fish parasitology. Fortunately, there are several proprietary anti-ectoparasite and anti-protozoan

> ### IMPORTANT
> **Never add new stock to an aquarium containing diseased fish. Wait at least four weeks after all symptoms of disease have gone before introducing new fish.**

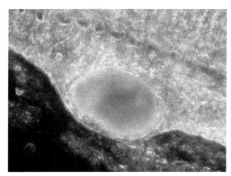

Skin irritation may affect a fish's gills. Pictured: whitespot parasite in gill tissue.

medications on the market that will kill a broad range of skin parasites.

The whole aquarium should be treated in order to destroy any free-living stages. One or two repeat treatments are usually required (check the manufacturer's instructions). Expert advice should be sought if the problem persists despite a full course of medication.

AQUARIUM INVADERS

The discovery of unusual worms or other creatures in the aquarium has often led the owner to believe that his tank is riddled with parasites. In fact, most visible 'free-roaming' creatures in the aquarium are harmless, the two common ones being planarian worms and copepods. As with snails, these creatures are brought in on plants or in the fish's transport water.

PLANARIAN WORMS

These small (2-10 mm) flat-worms may be seen gliding slowly over the aquarium surfaces and on the glass. There are several species that vary in colour from off-white, grey, brown to black. Their characteristic arrow-shaped heads may be seen with the aid of a magnifying lens.

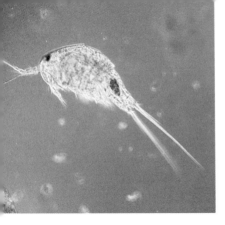

Large numbers of copepods in the aquarium may indicate poor aquarium hygiene.

COPEPODS

These tiny (to 3 mm) white to brown creatures may be seen attached to the glass and other surfaces, occasionally moving in a short hopping motion. A strong magnifying lens will reveal their tear-shaped body with two or more elongate hair-like appendages extending from their rear ends. They are more common in aquariums housing only large fish (small fish find them a delicacy!).

The presence of large numbers of planarians or copepods may indicate that the aquarium needs a spring-clean, as these creatures proliferate where there is lots of decaying organic matter in the aquarium.

Note: the only two fish parasites that may be seen freely in the aquarium are the fish louse (*Argulus*: disc-shaped, about 0.5-1cm in diameter) and the fish leech (*Piscicola*, which reaches several centimetres in length). However, both these parasites are extremely uncommon in tropical aquariums.

CHAPTER
5

DOSAGE AND TREATMENT

Most proprietary fish medications are sold in concentrated liquid form. These are diluted according to the manufacturer's instructions and added to the aquarium water. The fish are therefore immersed in a medication 'bath'.

When calculating the amount to dispense, you will need to know the water volume of the aquarium to be treated. It's a good idea to keep a record of the volume of your aquarium – expressed in both litres and gallons (see page 59 for calculating volume).

CALCULATING THE DOSE
Let's assume the medication is to be administered at 2 millilitres (ml) per gallon of water, and the aquarium holds 15 gallons. The amount to be dispensed is therefore 15 x 2 ml = 30 ml. Most commercial medications come with a measuring cap or vial, enabling a precise volume to be dispensed.

SAFETY CHECKS
- Be sure that you have correctly identified the disease and are using the most appropriate medication. Never experiment with a series of different medications in the hope that one may work.
- Never overdose. Most medications are slightly toxic to fish, such that overdosing can harm or even kill fish.

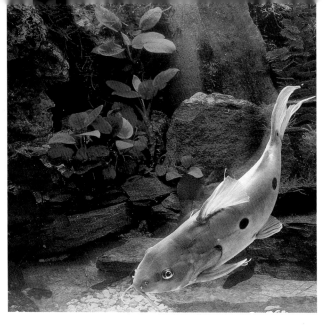

Most medications are slightly toxic to fish, so never overdose. Certainly catfish (pictured above) are particularly sensitive to some medications.

- Never use a combination of different medications unless professionally advised to do so. Certain mixtures may prove harmful to fish.
- Don't pour concentrated medication (i.e. straight from the bottle) into the aquarium. Mix first with a small amount of tap water in a clean cup or container. Accidental exposure to concentrated medication can be lethal to fish.
- Check whether the medication harms biological filtration. Some products contain chemicals that destroy the beneficial filter bacteria – look for warning notes on the manufacturer's instructions. If so, you will either have to isolate the filter during medication or wait for it to re-mature (i.e. recolonise with bacteria) after the course of treatment has finished.

- Take care when handling medications, especially in concentrated form. Some, such as formalin and malachite green, can be harmful to humans if used incorrectly. Check the manufacturer's instructions for any health warning signs. If in doubt about handling chemicals, wear clean, disposable gloves.
- With some diseases, it will be necessary to administer one or more repeat doses of medication, usually every few days (again, refer to the manufacturer's instructions).

TREATING FISH IN ISOLATION

Most medications are added to the whole aquarium. In some cases, however, it may be preferable to remove the sick fish to a hospital tank to treat them in isolation (see Quarantine, page 19 and 20). The manufacturer's instructions generally provide guidance in this respect.

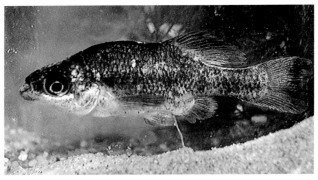

In some instances, fish should be isolated in a hospital tank to receive treatment. Pictured: A Mexican livebearing fish with emaciation and stringy faeces, possibly indicating an internal bacterial infection.

CHAPTER 6

EUTHANASIA

Despite all your best efforts, you may be faced with the prospect of having to 'put down' a badly diseased or injured fish for which there is little hope of recovery. Contrary to popular belief, fish *are* capable of experiencing pain and stress, and therefore must never be left to suffer unnecessarily.

The decision whether to euthanase a fish or keep it alive with the hope it gets better can be a difficult one

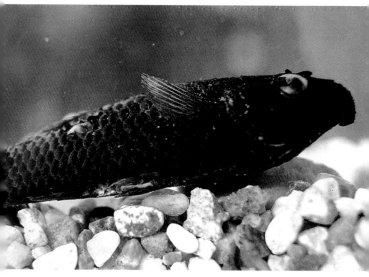

Contrary to popular belief, fish can experience pain, so, humane euthanasia should be practised quickly to end suffering, as in the case of this dying molly.

and you may feel more comfortable in seeking advice from the local aquarium store, an experienced aquarium hobbyist, or a veterinary surgeon.

ACCEPTABLE METHODS

The subject of fish euthanasia is often taboo in the aquarium literature, resulting in ignorance and unsuitable methods being practised.

Basically, there are two acceptable methods for killing a fish:

CONCUSSION

The fish is removed from the water and its body is wrapped in a sheet of soft paper tissue. The fish is then held on a firm solid surface (floor or strong table) and its exposed head is struck with a hard heavy object such as a hammer. This may seem barbaric, but is actually fast and effective. The aim is to destroy the fish's brain swiftly.

If you feel uneasy about performing this procedure then it is best not to do it: a half-hearted attempt may be unsuccessful and cause further suffering to the fish. Instead, find a competent aquarist who is less squeamish, or take the fish to a vet.

ANAESTHETIC OVERDOSE

Fish anaesthetics, such as MS222 and Benzocaine, can be administered at a lethal 'overdose' level. The fish is placed in a solution of anaesthetic until it loses consciousness and dies. This method is ideal for killing large numbers of fish and for specimens that are too big to be euthanased by concussion.

This procedure should only be undertaken by an

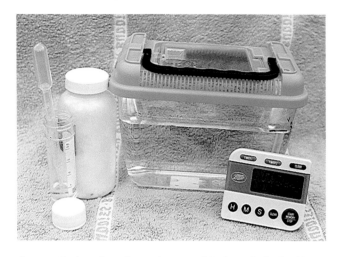

An anaesthetic tank used to euthanase a fish. Anaesthesia should only be performed by an experienced aquarist or vet.

experienced aquarist or vet as it requires skill to properly gauge the amount of anaesthetic required and to tell when the fish is actually dead.

In some countries, fish anaesthetics are obtainable legally only on veterinary prescription. Consult your aquarium store or vet regarding supplies and use.

UNSUITABLE METHODS
These will cause the fish considerable suffering and are completely unacceptable methods of euthanasia:
- Slow freezing by placing the fish (in a container of water) in a domestic freezer. Although still routinely practised by fishkeepers, it is now considered unacceptable.
- Dropping the fish into very hot/boiling water.
- Leaving the fish to die out of water.
- Snapping the fish's backbone.

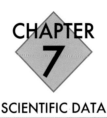

CHAPTER
7

SCIENTIFIC DATA

Conversions are given to two decimal places.

LENGTH
1 metre = 100 centimetres (cm)
1 centimetre = 10 millimetres (mm)
1 mm = 1000 microns (μm)
1 centimetre = 0.39 inches (in)
1 inch = 2.54 cm

WEIGHT
1 kilogram (kg) = 1000 grams (g)
1 gram = 1000 milligrams (mg)
1 milligram = 1000 micrograms (μg)
1 kg = 2.20 pounds (lbs)

VOLUME
1 litre = 1000 millilitres (ml/mL) = 1000 cubic cm (cm^3)
1 litre (l or L) = 0.22 imperial gallons*
1 imperial gallon = 4.55 litres
1 US gallon = 3.79 litres
1 cubic foot of water = 6.23 imperial gallons

* In the UK, the imperial system is used for gallons.

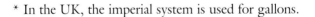

CONCENTRATIONS (e.g. for dosing with medications)

1 part per thousand (ppt) = 1 gram per litre
1 part per million (ppm) = 1 mg per litre

AQUARIUM CAPACITY AND WEIGHT

To calculate aquarium volume: multiply length x depth x width (in cm) to give volume in cubic centimetres (cm^3). Divide by 1000 to give the volume in litres.

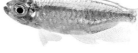

For example, an aquarium of dimensions 90 cm length, 30 cm depth, 30 cm width has a volume of 81,000 cm^3. Divide by 1000 = 81 litres (=17.8 imperial gallons).

One litre of water weighs 1 kg. Hence, a 81-litre aquarium can hold 81 kg (=178 lbs) of water.

AQUARIUM SURFACE AREA

Multiply aquarium length by width (in cm) to give its surface area in square centimetres (cm^2).

FISH STOCKING DENSITY

As a rule of thumb, allow 25 cm^2 surface area for every centimetre body length of fish (excluding tail). (Note: these calculations do not apply to coldwater or marine fish.)
For example, an aquarium of 100 cm length and 30 cm width has a surface area of 3000 cm^2. Thus, 3000 divided by 25 gives 125 =

total body length of fish, in cm. In this example, the tank can accommodate five 25-cm fish, ten 12.5-cm fish, etc., or combinations thereof. Important: use the fish's *adult* size when making these calculations, so the aquarium can safely accommodate the fish when fully grown.

TEMPERATURE

°C = degrees Centigrade (also known as Celsius)
°F = degrees Fahrenheit

Centigrade to Fahrenheit conversion (Fahrenheit values given to nearest degree):

°C	°F
0	32
5	41
10	50
20	68
21	70
22	72
23	73
24	75
25	77
26	79
27	81
28	82
29	84
30	86

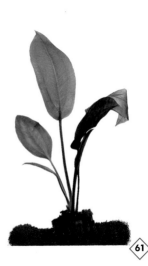

Acute: in reference to disease – sudden or fast-acting (cf. chronic).

Biotope: a habitat/environment and the living things contained within it.

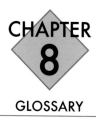

Chronic: in reference to disease – long-term or slow-acting (cf. acute).

Dechlorinated/dechlorination: removal of chlorine.

Ectoparasites: parasites that live on the fish's body surface (as opposed to endoparasites that live inside).

Fin-nipping: certain fish have a reputation for biting the fins of others, and the victims are vulnerable to fin infections. Fish that constantly fin-nip must be removed from the aquarium.

Flashing: the fish turns on its side to rub its flanks against a firm object, such as a rock or gravel. Repeated flashing is often a sign of adverse water conditions or skin parasites.

Free-living stage: the stage of a parasite that lives off the fish. Some parasites have two or more free-living stages. cf. Parasitic stage.

Haemorrhage: bleeding caused by loss of blood from the blood vessels.

Life cycle: usually in reference to parasites that pass through various stages in order to complete one generation. The life cycles of some fish parasites are complex and may involve the sequential infection of a fish, a land animal (e.g. a bird) and an aquatic invertebrate, such as a freshwater shrimp or snail.

Optimum (aquarium) conditions: husbandry conditions that best suit the fish species in question. Conditions include water chemistry and temperature, diet, lighting, aquarium décor, substrate, and suitability of tankmates.

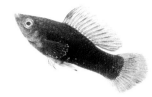

Parasitic stage: the stage of a parasite that lives on or within the fish's body. cf. Free-living stage.

Pathogen: an organism that causes disease.